HERBS FOR CROHN'S DISEASE

Healing Harvest, Unlocking Nature's Remedies For Stress Relief

DR. JEREMY ALLEY

Disclaimer:

The information provided in this book, is intended for general informational purposes only and should not be considered as professional advice.

The author has made every effort to ensure the accuracy of the information presented. However, readers are advised to consult with a qualified healthcare professional before attempting any herbal remedies or making significant changes to their wellness routine. Individual health conditions vary, and what may be suitable for one person may not be appropriate for another.

It is important to note that the author is not in any endorsement deal, partnership, or affiliation with any organization, brand, or company mentioned in this book. Any references to specific products or services are based on the author's personal experience or general knowledge and do not imply an endorsement or promotion of those products or services.

Contents

Overview

Crohn's disease is a chronic inflammatory ailment that can greatly affect a person's quality of life, making it difficult to live with. Even though traditional medical care is essential for controlling Crohn's disease, many people look for supplementary methods to reduce symptoms and enhance their general health. Herbal treatments are becoming more and more well-liked as an additional choice for treating Crohn's disease symptoms. This book tries to offer helpful insights into combining these natural interventions into an all-encompassing wellness plan by examining the significance of herbal remedies in treating the difficulties caused by Crohn's disease.

Concerning Crohn's Disease

One form of inflammatory bowel disease (IBD) that is distinguished by persistent gastrointestinal tract inflammation is Crohn's disease. Any portion of the digestive system, from the mouth to the anus, can be affected, and symptoms like diarrhea, exhaustion, weight loss, and abdominal discomfort can result. The precise etiology of Crohn's disease is yet unknown, however, it frequently results from a complex interaction between the immune system, environmental, and genetic variables. Medications, lifestyle changes, and, in extreme situations, surgery are the usual therapies for Crohn's disease. However, many people are investigating herbal medicines as a way to manage symptoms and support digestive health as a result of their search for complementary and alternative ways.

The Function of Herbal Treatments

For ages, a variety of traditional medicinal systems have employed herbal remedies to treat a broad range of illnesses, including digestive issues. Certain herbs are thought to have anti-inflammatory, antibacterial, and immune-modulating qualities that may help with Crohn's disease symptom relief. Herbs having anti-inflammatory properties, such as aloe vera, Boswellia, and turmeric, may help reduce the inflammation brought on by Crohn's disease. Herbal medicines like ginger, peppermint, and chamomile may also help with digestive problems including bloating and pain in the abdomen. Anyone thinking about using herbal therapies as part of their care plan for Crohn's disease must be aware of the possible advantages and disadvantages of doing so.

How This Book Can Be Useful

This book is a thorough reference for anyone looking for information on herbal treatments for Crohn's disease. It looks at the historical background of particular plants in traditional medicine, their putative mechanisms of action, and the science underlying their use. The practical aspects of integrating herbal therapies into daily life will become clearer to readers as they take into account things like dose, preparation techniques, and potential drug interactions. Furthermore, the book offers a fair-minded viewpoint by stressing the available scientific data and dispelling myths about herbal treatments for Crohn's disease. This book seeks to improve readers' ability to make informed decisions and improve the general well-being of people with Crohn's disease by arming them with knowledge.

CHAPTER ONE

RECOGNIZING CRONENBERG'S ILLNESS

An inflammatory bowel disease (IBD) that can affect any section of the digestive tract is called Crohn's disease. It is a chronic condition. Deeply rooted inflammation that penetrates the lining of the impacted intestinal tissue is its defining feature. Different from ulcerative colitis, which affects only the colon, Crohn's disease affects the entire digestive tract, extending from the mouth to the anus. Although the precise origin of Crohn's disease is still unknown, a mix of immune system, environmental, and genetic variables are thought to be involved.

Crohn's Disease: What Is It?

The intricate and persistent ailment known as Crohn's disease arises from the immune system of the body inadvertently targeting healthy cells within the digestive system. Crohn's disease-related inflammation can cause a variety of symptoms, such as exhaustion and weight loss in addition to diarrhea and abdominal pain. Individual differences in the degree and location of inflammation contribute to the disease's unpredictability and difficulty in management.

Signs And Prognosis

Crohn's disease frequently manifests as diarrhea, exhaustion, decreased appetite, weight loss, and abdominal pain. Nonetheless, every person may uniquely experience the illness.

A combination of imaging procedures (such as endoscopy and colonoscopy), physical examination, medical history assessment, and laboratory testing is usually used to provide a diagnosis. A healthcare provider must be consulted to receive an accurate diagnosis and a suitable treatment plan.

Reasons And Initiators

Although the precise causes of Crohn's disease are unknown, several factors related to the immune system, environment, and heredity are thought to play a role. Genetics are involved because those who have a family history of IBD are more likely to develop the disease. Environmental elements may also have a role, including nutrition, smoking, and contact with specific microorganisms. Identifying and controlling triggers—such as stress and particular foods—can be essential to symptom management.

Effects On Day-To-Day Living

A person's everyday life can be greatly impacted by having Crohn's disease. The disease's unpredictable nature combined with symptoms including frequent toilet breaks and abdominal pain can make it difficult to work, interact with others, and carry out daily tasks. For those with Crohn's disease, managing the psychological and emotional effects of having a chronic illness is crucial to their overall well-being.

Traditional Methods Of Treatment

The goals of traditional Crohn's disease therapies are to lessen inflammation, manage symptoms, and enhance quality of life. To treat the illness, medical experts usually use a mix of prescription drugs and sometimes surgery. To choose the best course of treatment for their unique requirements, people with Crohn's disease must collaborate closely with their medical team.

Drugs

Many kinds of drugs are frequently used to treat Crohn's disease. Among the alternatives are biologics, immunosuppressants, and anti-inflammatory medications. Anti-inflammatory medications, like aminosalicylates and corticosteroids, aid in the reduction of inflammation. Immunosuppressants function by reducing the activity of the immune system, such as methotrexate and azathioprine. Certain inflammatory pathways are targeted by biologics like adalimumab and infliximab. The location and severity of the disease determine which drug is best.

Procedures

Surgery may be an option if the medicine is not working or if complications develop. Reconnecting healthy sections of the digestive tract, removing the diseased piece, or constructing a stoma are surgical procedures for Crohn's disease.

Generally speaking, surgery is only performed under certain circumstances, and the choice to have surgery is taken after consulting a medical specialist.

Although Crohn's disease can be effectively managed with drugs and surgery, there is a possibility that these treatments will have negative effects. People must be informed about the potential dangers and advantages of each available treatment choice. An elevated risk of infections, exhaustion, and nausea are typical adverse effects. To provide the best possible outcome for the patient with Crohn's disease, healthcare providers carefully consider the benefits of treatment about probable adverse effects.

CHAPTER TWO

OVERVIEW OF HERBAL REMEDIES

Throughout history, herbal remedies have played a vital role in traditional medicine by providing a comprehensive approach to treating a wide range of illnesses. The usage of herbs has drawn attention due to its therapeutic benefits in the setting of Crohn's disease, an inflammatory bowel illness that affects the digestive tract. Examining the historical foundations of herbs as well as the increasing amount of scientific data proving their effectiveness is essential to comprehending their power.

Herbs' Power

For millennia, medicinal methods have relied heavily on herbs in many different civilizations. Herbs' abundance of plant-based chemicals offers a wide range of possible health advantages. Numerous herbs include anti-inflammatory, antibacterial, and antioxidant qualities that can help with the treatment of long-term illnesses like Crohn's disease. Recognizing the complex interactions between the natural components of herbs and their effects on the human body is essential to maximizing their power.

Use In The Past

Herbal treatments for digestive problems, such as Crohn's disease-like illnesses, have long been used in traditional medicine.

To treat digestive problems, traditional medical systems such as Ayurveda, Traditional Chinese medicine, and Native American medicine have used particular herbs.

This historical background sheds important light on the long-held notion that herbs are effective in supporting digestive health and treating inflammatory diseases.

Despite the strong historical evidence, the scientific world is focusing more and more on proving the efficacy of herbal medicines.

The identification and comprehension of the bioactive substances found in herbs, as well as their mechanisms of action, have been made possible by modern research approaches. Research on the anti-inflammatory, antioxidative, and immunomodulatory properties of specific herbs helps to establish the scientific basis for incorporating herbal medicines into the treatment of Crohn's disease.

Categories Of Herbal Remedies

It is easier to streamline the possible benefits of herbal therapies for Crohn's disease by classifying them. Herbs that promote gut healing, inhibit inflammation, and alter the immune system fall into three main categories.

Reducing Inflammation Herbs

Herbs that reduce inflammation are an important class in treating Crohn's disease symptoms. Certain herbs, like Boswellia serrata, ginger, and turmeric, have shown anti-inflammatory properties that may help reduce the disease's chronic inflammation. These herbs may lessen the intensity of symptoms and block inflammatory pathways, offering an alternative to traditional treatments.

Herbs For Gut Healing

When it comes to managing Crohn's disease, the gastrointestinal tract's integrity is crucial. Some plants, such as marshmallow root, aloe vera, and slippery elm, are prized for their calming qualities and high mucilage content.

These herbs may support general gut health and aid in symptom relief by protecting and mending the lining of the digestive tract.

Immune-Suppressive Herbs

Immunomodulating herbs provide a focused strategy, considering the immune system's role in the development of Crohn's disease. Herbs that modify immune responses, such as reishi mushrooms, astragalus, and echinacea, may help prevent excessive inflammation and improve immunological balance.

The goal of including these herbs in a thorough treatment regimen is to address the immunological dysregulation that underlies Crohn's disease.

Herbal treatments for Crohn's disease offer a comprehensive method of managing symptoms. Herbs have long been used, and there is mounting scientific evidence to support their potential advantages when used in a full treatment strategy.

Comprehending the classifications of anti-inflammatory, gut-healing, and immune-modulating herbs facilitates a customized strategy that corresponds with the intricate characteristics of Crohn's disease.

As with any medical problem, seeking professional advice is necessary to guarantee the safe and efficient incorporation of herbal treatments into the overall treatment plan.

CHAPTER THREE

ESTABLISHING A BASIS

Nutrition And Diet

Nutrition is a key component of Crohn's disease management, and establishing a nutrient-dense, well-balanced diet is critical to establishing general wellness. Nutrient absorption is frequently problematic for Crohn's disease sufferers, therefore it's critical to emphasize foods that are quickly digested and easy on the digestive tract.

Foods Suitable For Crohn's

Including items that are Crohn's disease-friendly in your diet is essential for treating the condition. These consist of foods that are simple to digest, like cooked grains, lean meats, and fruits and vegetables. Including foods high in omega-3 fatty acids, such as fish and flaxseeds, may also have anti-inflammatory properties that could help with symptom control.

Items To Steer Clear Of

A key component of nutritional treatment is recognizing and avoiding trigger foods, which can aggravate Crohn's disease symptoms.

Dairy products, fried or greasy foods, high-fiber fruits and vegetables, and spicy foods are common triggers. Maintaining a food journal enables people to identify particular foods that can exacerbate symptoms, enabling a more individualized approach to food selection.

Supplements For Nutrition

Supplemental nutrition can be very helpful in ensuring that vital vitamin and mineral levels remain at an appropriate level when there is a problem with nutrient absorption. Healthcare providers may provide supplements including vitamin D, iron, and B vitamins to treat deficiencies and promote general health.

Modifications In Lifestyle

Making healthy lifestyle choices can have a big impact on how Crohn's disease is managed. Giving up smoking is a crucial lifestyle change because smoking has been connected to an increased risk of flare-ups. For those with Crohn's disease, drinking alcohol in moderation and maintaining hydration are also essential components of a healthy lifestyle.

Stress Reduction

It is well-recognized that stress can precipitate or worsen Crohn's disease symptoms. Using stress-reduction methods like yoga, deep breathing exercises, and mindfulness meditation can help to improve both mental and physical health. For people with Crohn's disease, creating a customized stress management strategy is crucial to reducing the negative effects of stress on their illness.

Physical Activity And Exercise

Frequent exercise can be very helpful for those with Crohn's disease and has been demonstrated to have positive benefits on general health. Moderate activity, like cycling, swimming, or walking, can strengthen the immune system, aid in reducing inflammation, and enhance digestion. It's crucial to confer with medical experts to create an exercise program that suits each person's requirements and capabilities.

Hygiene Of Sleep

The general health of people with Crohn's disease depends on getting enough good sleep. Inadequate sleep might worsen symptoms and impair immunological response.

For people with Crohn's disease, establishing appropriate sleep hygiene practices—such as keeping a regular sleep schedule, setting up a cozy sleeping environment, and abstaining from stimulants before bed—can improve both the quality of their sleep and general health.

CHAPTER FOUR

ESSENTIAL HERBAL CURES

Managing Crohn's disease, a chronic inflammatory bowel disease, can be difficult. While there are traditional therapies available, some people look into herbal remedies to help with symptoms and general health. We examine important choices such as marshmallow root, slippery elm, aloe vera, turmeric and curcumin, and aloe vera in this investigation of herbal treatments for Crohn's disease.

Qualities And Advantages

Curcumin, the key ingredient in turmeric, a bright yellow spice derived from the Curcuma longa plant, has drawn interest. Because of its anti-inflammatory and antioxidant qualities, curcumin may be useful in treating the symptoms of Crohn's disease. It might assist in regulating the immune system and lowering gastrointestinal inflammation.

Dosage & Setting Up

Different dosages of supplements containing turmeric or curcumin are advised. A healthcare provider should be consulted to determine the proper dosage based on each person's needs. There are several kinds of turmeric supplements on the market, such as powders, pills, and teas. Some people choose to add turmeric to food as a tasty and healthful way to increase their intake of the spice.

Calming Impacts On The Intestine

Well-known for its calming qualities, aloe vera has been suggested as a possible aid in treating Crohn's disease symptoms.

Aloe vera leaf gel is made up of substances that have healing and anti-inflammatory qualities. These characteristics might help lessen gastrointestinal tract irritation and inflammation.

CHAPTER FIVE

UTILIZATION AND APPLICATION

Aloe vera can be taken as supplements or in juice form, among other ways. Selecting premium, pure aloe vera products is crucial to guaranteeing both efficacy and safety.

Aloe vera has been shown to provide relief for some people; nevertheless, it is important to monitor its effects and get medical advice before using it regularly.

Mucilage Concentration

Derived from the inner bark of the Ulmus rubra tree, slippery elm has a lot of mucilage, which is a gel-like material with calming effects.

The mucilage found in slippery elm may coat and shield the digestive tract, which may lessen Crohn's disease symptoms.

Methods Of Preparation

Slippery elm comes in a variety of forms, such as powders, capsules, and teas. Some people like to combine the powder with water to make a slippery elm gruel. It creates a calming, easily absorbed solution that is ingested to offer comfort. It is essential to speak with a healthcare provider to ascertain the proper dosage and preparation technique for any herbal medicine.

Healing And Protective Qualities

The plant Althaea officinalis yields marshmallow root, which is prized for having a mucilaginous quality akin to that of slippery elm.

The digestive tract may benefit from the preventive and restorative properties of marshmallow root mucilage, which may lessen Crohn's disease symptoms.

There are several types of marshmallow root available, such as tinctures, teas, and capsules. To experience the calming benefits of marshmallow root tea, some people prefer to consume it.

Including marshmallow root in your daily regimen could require speaking with a medical expert to figure out the best dosage and type for you.

Herbal treatments such as marshmallow root, slippery elm, aloe vera, turmeric, and curcumin show the potential to help people with Crohn's disease.

To ensure safety and efficacy in specific circumstances, it is imperative to exercise caution when utilizing these cures and to speak with healthcare professionals.

Developing Customized Herbal Plans

Making customized herbal regimens is often beneficial for those looking for herbal therapies for Crohn's disease. These plans take into account the patient's particular situation, symptoms, and general health. Patients can increase the efficacy of their management techniques by customizing herbal therapies to meet their unique requirements.

Meeting with a Herbalist

Speak with an experienced herbalist before creating a customized herbal regimen for Crohn's disease. Professionals with training in the use of medicinal plants to enhance health and treat specific conditions are known as herbalists. The herbalist collects data from the patient during consultation regarding their symptoms, medical background, and way of life to formulate a customized and all-encompassing approach to Crohn's disease management.

CHAPTER SIX

LOCATING AN ACCREDITED PROFESSIONAL

For anyone looking into herbal therapies for Crohn's disease, finding a certified herbal practitioner is crucial. It is best to look for practitioners who have accreditation from respected herbalism institutions or pertinent professional associations, among other recognized credentials. Patients can put their trust in the skills and knowledge required to create an herbal treatment plan that is both safe and successful by selecting a certified practitioner.

What To Anticipate

Patients should anticipate a comprehensive conversation about their dietary practices, lifestyle, medical treatments currently under consideration, and symptoms of Crohn's disease during a consultation with a herbalist. Additionally, the herbalist could ask about any possible sensitivities, allergies, or other medical issues. This thorough investigation aids the herbalist in developing a comprehensive picture of the patient's health, which makes it possible to design a customized herbal regimen.

Creating A Herbal Protocol

After the first visit, the herbalist creates a customized herbal regimen for Crohn's disease management. This program could involve a mix of certain herbs, nutritional advice, lifestyle modifications, and possibly other holistic methods. Promoting general wellbeing and treating the underlying causes of Crohn's disease symptoms are the objectives.

The herbal treatment is intended to be practical and flexible enough to fit into the patient's everyday routine.

Customizing For Every Need

Herbal medicines are advantageous since they can be tailored to meet specific needs. The patient's individual qualities, including their constitution, temperament, and any coexisting medical issues, are taken into account by the herbalist. This customization guarantees that the herbal protocol is in harmony with the patient's body and raises the treatment's general efficacy. The herbal regimen may need to be modified in response to the patient's response and advancement.

Tracking Development

One of the most important aspects of using herbal medicines for Crohn's disease is to regularly assess the patient's development. Herbalists collaborate extensively with patients to evaluate how the herbal treatment affects their symptoms, energy, digestion, and general health. This continuous partnership makes it possible to modify the herbal plan as needed, keeping it efficient and in line with the patient's changing medical requirements. Together, the patient and the herbalist monitor the patient's development, encouraging a comprehensive and individualized approach to using herbal treatments to manage Crohn's disease.

CHAPTER SEVEN

SUCCESS STORIES AND CASE STUDIES

Actual Experiences

Living with Crohn's disease can be difficult, but using herbal medicines has helped some people find relief and progress in their condition. These success stories and case studies offer insightful information about the experiences of patients who successfully managed their Crohn's disease using herbal remedies.

Patient A: Managing Outbursts

The experience of Patient A with Crohn's disease was characterized by frequent flare-ups and a quest for efficient symptom control. After experiencing no improvement with traditional therapy, Patient A looked into using herbal remedies as a substitute. Patient A saw a significant improvement in the frequency and intensity of flare-ups as well as a reduction in inflammation thanks to a well-chosen herbal combination that included aloe vera, Boswellia, and turmeric. This case study provides insight into the possible advantages of using herbal remedies to treat acute Crohn's disease symptoms.

Patient B: Long-Term Symptom Management

Maintaining a high quality of life and long-term symptom control were the key goals for Patient B. While some alleviation was obtained from traditional pharmaceuticals, Patient B looked into herbal alternatives due to worries about possible adverse effects. The daily regimen that included marshmallow root, chamomile, and slippery elm produced long-lasting improvements in overall health and digestive health. The experience of Patient B highlights the value of herbal treatments in offering a comprehensive and long-lasting method of managing Crohn's disease.

Crohn's Disease Remedies Made With Herbs

Ginger

Due to its anti-inflammatory qualities and active ingredient curcumin, turmeric is a popular choice among people with Crohn's disease. According to studies, turmeric may be able to lessen digestive tract inflammation and ease symptoms including diarrhea and abdominal pain.

Boswellia

Because of its anti-inflammatory qualities, Boswellia, which is derived from the resin of the Boswellia tree, has been utilized in traditional medicine. After adding boswellia to their treatment plan, some Crohn's disease patients have experienced improvements in symptoms like diarrhea and stomach pain.

Vera Aloe

Known for its calming qualities, aloe vera may be beneficial for those who suffer from Crohn's disease. Aloe vera may aid in gastrointestinal tract inflammation reduction and mucosal lining healing, according to certain research.

Slippery Elm

Slippery elm is frequently applied topically to relieve inflamed gastrointestinal system tissues. When combined with water, it creates a gel-like substance that can coat the intestinal lining to protect it. This can be especially helpful for people who have Crohn's disease and are having ulceration and inflammation.

Chamomile

Due to its relaxing properties, chamomile may help relieve Crohn's disease symptoms like cramping and stomach pain. Because of its anti-inflammatory and anti-spasmodic qualities, it could be used as an adjunctive treatment.

Marshmallow Root

Because of its mucilaginous qualities, marshmallow root is thought to coat the lining of the digestive tract in protection.

As a result, people with Crohn's disease may experience relief from their irritation and inflammation.

Herbal treatments have the potential to help control Crohn's disease symptoms, but before implementing these options into a treatment plan, people should speak with medical professionals.

Though each person's experience with Crohn's disease is different, and what works for one person may not work for another, case studies and success stories offer insightful tales. Herbal medicines may provide more options for people looking for symptom alleviation when incorporated within a complete and individualized approach to managing Crohn's disease.

CHAPTER EIGHT

COMBINING HERBAL REMEDIES WITH TRADITIONAL MEDICATION

A chronic inflammatory bowel disease that can seriously lower a person's quality of life is Crohn's disease. While medicine and surgery are the most popular forms of traditional medical treatment, some people look into complementary and alternative therapies, such as herbal remedies, to manage their symptoms. It is imperative to approach the cautious and cooperative integration of herbal therapies with conventional treatments.

Working Together With Medical Professionals

It's important to speak with medical experts, such as gastroenterologists, naturopathic physicians, and herbalists, before using herbal therapies to treat Crohn's disease. By utilizing collaborative decision-making, possible risks are reduced and all elements of the treatment plan are taken into account. Depending on the patient's medical history and the severity of Crohn's disease, healthcare professionals can provide important information on the safety and effectiveness of particular herbal therapies.

Techniques Of Communication

When evaluating herbal medicines in addition to conventional treatments, individuals and healthcare professionals must communicate openly and honestly. Patients should disclose to their medical team any information regarding any herbal supplements they are taking or intend to use, including dosage and frequency information.

 On the other hand, to guarantee that patients fully comprehend their treatment plan, medical professionals should make sure to ask about patients' use of herbal remedies during routine checkups.

Observing And Modifying

Integrating herbal therapies requires careful monitoring of illness progression and symptoms regularly. Patients and medical staff need to collaborate to monitor any changes in symptoms and modify treatment plans as necessary. This could entail altering the amount or kind of herbal remedies taken, as well as taking into account any possible negative reactions or side effects.

Possible Relationships And Things To Think About

The efficacy or safety of conventional drugs or other therapies may be affected by interactions between herbal remedies. It is critical to take into account these possible interconnections and base judgments on the unique circumstances of each individual. To reduce any negative effects, factors such as the patient's overall health, current drugs, and Crohn's disease stage should be carefully considered.

Interference With Medication

Some herbal therapies have the potential to hinder the efficacy or absorption of prescribed Crohn's disease drugs. Herbs such as St John's wort can stimulate liver enzymes, which can impact how certain medications are metabolized. To guarantee that patients benefit fully from both conventional pharmaceuticals and herbal therapies, healthcare providers should be on the lookout for potential conflicts and modify treatment plans accordingly.

Taking Care of Safety

When using herbal medicines for Crohn's disease treatment, safety is crucial.

Healthcare providers must educate patients with adequate information regarding the potential hazards and advantages of herbal supplements, so they may make informed and safe decisions. Furthermore, as variations in product composition might affect the safety and effectiveness of the product, it is imperative to purchase herbal goods from reliable suppliers to guarantee quality and purity.

It takes teamwork and knowledge to combine herbal treatments with traditional Crohn's disease care. A thorough treatment plan that takes into account the specific requirements of each patient with Crohn's disease can be developed by healthcare professionals and patients by encouraging open communication, keeping an eye on symptoms, and taking possible interactions into account. Those dealing with this difficult illness may benefit from better symptom management and general well-being as a result of this comprehensive approach.

FINAL VERDICT

Investigating herbal treatments for Crohn's disease might be a decision that each individual makes to better control symptoms and enhance general health. It's critical to approach these treatments with knowledge, taking into account specific medical issues and seeking advice from medical experts.

Summary Of Important Ideas

For those looking for information about herbal therapies for Crohn's disease, this section provides a short reference that highlights the main ideas covered in the previous sections.

Motivation For The Upcoming Trip

Crohn's disease can be difficult to live with, but it's crucial to maintain your optimism and concentrate on symptom management. Encouragement is provided in this part, which highlights the value of a comprehensive strategy that incorporates lifestyle modifications, medical treatments, and if preferred, supplemental herbal therapies.

 Even though the road may include ups and downs, people with Crohn's disease can strive for a higher quality of life with the correct assistance and guidance.

www.ingramcontent.com/pod-product-compliance
Lightning Source LLC
Chambersburg PA
CBHW060845260726
48661CB00002B/621